The Insiders Guide to Hiring A World-Class Dental Team

A Revolutionary Approach To Recruiting,
Hiring, Training, and Retaining
World-Class Dental Professionals

JOHN J. MEIS
WENDY BRIGGS

THE TEAM TRAINING INSTITUTE

THE INSIDERS GUIDE TO HIRING A WORLD-CLASS DENTAL TEAM:
A REVULOUTIONARY APPROACH TO RECRUITING, HIRING, TRAINING, AND
RETAINING WORLD-CLASS DENTAL PROFESSIONALS

MEIS, JOHN J.
BRIGGS, WENDY

ISBN 978-0692676059

THE TEAM TRAINING INSTITUTE
12 W 100 N, SUITE 102, AMERICAN FORK, UT 84003 - U.S.A.
WWW.THETEAMTRAININGINSTITUTE.COM
(877) 732-2124

ACKNOWLEDGMENTS

We wish to thank our families for their love and support without which, our work and this book would not be possible.

We wish to thank the wonderful people on our team who helped bring this project to fruition:

Heather Driscoll - for the many contributions in terms of ideas, concepts, theories, and her overall common sense.

Austin Granzow - for endless hours spent formatting and editing this book.

Heidi Oligmueller - for her guidance and wisdom on employment legal matters.

Finally, we would be remiss if we did not also acknowledge the contributions of Brenda Goude, Brad May, Camie Schoonover, Cathy Ariana, Tara Hart, Karrie O'Neill, Kristie Kapp, Bertha Triche, Laurie Kimball, and Jeff Goude.

John J. Meis

Wendy Briggs

Table of Contents

Overview of the X Factor Series

This book explores how to build your own dental dream team.

The problems with building a dental team are so pervasive. "How can we build our team?" and "How can we have a great team?" are the two most common questions we are asked.

When we first studied big and successful practices, we noticed they all had really great teams. We had thought it was because of their size and success that they were able to attract these wonderful teams, but we had it backwards. They became great practices because they had wonderful teams and wonderful leaders. The leadership helped their teams get better and better.

We're going to share with you how you can build the best dental team. We'll cover the nuts and bolts of how to go from where you are now to having the kind of team you have only dreamed of.

The Cost of a Bad Hire

When the team building process goes wrong, it goes really wrong.

- Today, 1 in 5 civil lawsuits are filed by a current or a former employee.

- Employees make up 20% of all lawsuits.

- The cost of a bad hire is 150%–300% of their annual salary for each year that they are employed.

Imagine having a bad hire who has worked for you for two years. Let's say it's a dental assistant who makes $40,000/year; this means that the potential cost of that hire not working out is $120,000.

At any given time, 15% of practices are in some kind of crisis mode. In fact, one common crisis is being in litigation. Litigation is difficult. It's heart-wrenching. It's anxiety producing. It can drain an awful lot of hard work and effort in a very short amount of time.

Dr. Meis:

When my kids were little and they wanted something expensive, I would say, "You want that? That's how much?"

Then I'd say, "That's a lot of fillings."

Of course, they all laugh about it now. I don't think I would say that to my kids today. I'd want them to have more of an abundance mentality. At the time, that was where my head was, so that's why I said, "$120,000. That's a lot of fillings."

Fundamentals of Team Building

Get It, Want It and Can Do It

Gino Wickman's *Traction: Get a Grip on Your Business* has the absolute best management and meeting structure for small businesses.

In the book, Wickman argues that teams should possess these three qualities:

1. **Get It.** They understand what you're trying to accomplish. We've all had team members who just didn't understand critical concepts. They didn't understand great customer service or teamwork, for instance.

2. **Want It.** They want success bad enough to do what has to be done. We've all experienced employees who have uninvolved attitudes similar to this: "Well, I'm here 8 to 5. I'll clock in and I'll clock out, but I'm not going to put any extra effort into this. It's not worth my time. I just don't want it that badly."

2. **Can Do It.** They are capable of doing the job well. Employees that can't do it are very difficult to deal with because they understand what you're trying to do, and

they want to do it. However, they just aren't capable of doing it.

You need to create a team that gets it, wants it and can do it.

Dr. Meis:

We experienced this with a team member that we all really liked, but she just couldn't do it. She made so many errors that we had to make a move. It was very hard on everyone.

The "Warm Body" Syndrome

A "warm body" is an employee who is physically there but who is not engaged. That employee either doesn't get it, doesn't want it or can't do it (or a combination of those three).

Loss of Productivity

When you have a "warm body" employee, you have an absolute loss of productivity. The problem is that you usually won't recognize it as lost productivity. You just wish they would "get on track."

A "warm body" brings all kinds of problems and errors. Important tasks are usually undone or done poorly. If such an employee doesn't get it, want it or can do it, expect a series of errors.

Loss of Patient Relationships

With a "warm body" in the team, you're going to lose relationships with your patients.

Whether they're verbal about it or not, patients can sense that an employee isn't engaged. When patients aren't receiving a world-class experience in your practice, expect a deterioration in your relationship with patients as they become distant over time.

Well-formed patient relationships can handle a few mistakes and a few ups and downs, but if this continues, the relationship with the patient suffers. Eventually, they'll form a relationship with another practice.

Management Time Under Short Supply

In every growing practice, management time and talent is frequently in short supply.

When you have these "warm bodies" walking around your practice in a zombie-like state, it takes up a lot of management's time, effort and energy to keep them motivated.
Employees should "come with batteries included." In other words, they should be self-motivated. You want them to be at work, follow systems, and if they see something that doesn't work, they'll figure out how they can improve it.

Dr. Meis:
I recently worked with the management team of a very large practice that had about 60 locations.

Their biggest challenge moving forward was not getting enough patients nor was it having enough dentistry to do.

It was having enough management time and talent to take care of all the things that needed to be done.

Low Morale

When you have someone who is not performing at the level of other team members, it causes morale to suffer.

Other employees may soon say, "Well, if she gets away with X, Y and Z, then maybe I can, too." It ends up bugging everyone. You won't know it right away because the deterioration of morale starts slowly and eats its way in.

It becomes crystal clear when that "warm body" employee is let go because all of a sudden morale jumps. You'll then realize that you didn't have a real team member, you just had a "warm body."

All in all, the "warm body" syndrome costs you a lot of time and money.

Handling "Warm Body" Issues

We'll show you how to avoid hiring a "warm body."

If you already have a "warm body," we'll show you how to give that employee every development opportunity to grow.

If you can't get them to develop into a high-functioning team member, we'll discuss the safest and most effective ways to make a separation.

Recruiting Employees

An understaffed practice, that's always one team member shy, is a common problem.

Often, it's not by choice. It's often thrust upon them when employees leave the practice for a variety of reasons: pregnancy, injury, illness, moving out of town, or they simply don't work out as team members.

Constantly Recruiting

Our practice and team members have a "we're always hiring" mindset.

The practice may not have a current position open, but if we find people we like, we make sure that we stay in contact with them so that when we do have open positions, we can offer a position to them.

Diagnosing the Need

Determine if you need additional help, and never wait until you see a gaping hole in the team to fill it. This capacity issue can be so subtle, you don't even know it's happening.

We challenge you to look at the opportunities you miss each day. For example:

- Are you passing up same-day treatment on patients?

- Are you always running late?

- Is the phone not being answered?

Use missed opportunities as a diagnosis tool to determine if you're short staffed.

Dr. Meis:

I can't tell you how many times I've called a practice during business hours, and I was not be able to get a live person on the phone. That absolutely blows my mind.

That's a great example of an understaffed practice; maybe by choice, maybe not.

Either way, it's a drainer on productivity and profitability.

Incentivizing Staff Referrals

As the saying goes, "Birds of a feather flock together."

Great team members are associated with other great people. Let them know you may not have a specific job opening today but that you're constantly looking for good people.

Our staff is incentivized to identify people they think would make a good fit at our practice and encourage them to apply for jobs openings.

If we hire someone they referred to our practice, they get a $600 bounty:

- $300 is given when the person is hired.

- $300 is given when their 90-day training period is completed.

It is split in half to ensure the new employee is both adequately trained and will stick around.

Rewarding our team for sending good people our way has been extremely successful for us.

Soliciting Great Employees in Other Businesses

Watch for people who are employees in other businesses, not just dental practices, who have a great customer service attitude: Employees who are friendly, warm and sharp.

Leave your business card with such people and say, "We don't have any openings right now, but if you wouldn't mind sending your resume, we'll let you know when we do. I think you'd be a great addition to our team."

You won't know if they're looking for another opportunity or another experience until you ask. They may not be happy in their current position.

Whether they're interested or not, people are really flattered when you say that. Besides, there's no harm done by putting out feelers to see if they're looking for another career opportunity.

Advertising a Position

We'll occasionally advertise an open position in addition to these methods. This is very rare, but we do it once in a while.

Sometimes, we'll also notify local community colleges and unemployment agencies when we're looking to hire.

Career Opportunity Night

When we have an opening, hosting a career opportunity night is the first thing we do to narrow down our list of potential employees.

What people dread so much about the traditional hiring process is the time and decisions involved in picking employees based on resumes:

- Who will be the best three or seven applicants to interview?

- Should they come back for a second interview?

- Should they meet the team?

We fast-forward through all of that. We take this pipeline of people we're constantly cultivating and invite them to a career opportunity night.

We bring everyone together on a night after the practice has closed. This is so much more effective than spending long hours interviewing (which is grueling for both the applicant and the interviewer). It also allows you to skip over all of the basic first impression aspects that are usually done one-on-one.

Selling Applicants on Your Practice and the Position

Career Opportunity Night always includes a sales pitch on why we think our practice is great.

It's an opportunity to create a great deal of desire for people wanting to work in our practice. We talk about all the fun activities we do as a team, including community involvement and charity events. We talk about our greater social purpose.

Most importantly, we sell them on the available position and tell them:

- Why it's a great position.

- Why someone will want to have that position.

- Why it's so much fun.

- Why are practices such a great place to work.

We also sell potential applicants on the fact that our practice is growing. Things are always changing, so there's always going to be greater opportunities and chances for skills development.

We talk about the things that people may not like, too. For many people, our practice doesn't have very desirable hours. We start early in the morning; we see our first patient at 7 A.M. We're also there one night a week until 7 P.M.

Although we tell potential applicants upfront about all the good, bad and ugly elements of the position, we mainly focus on the good because we're really trying to sell them on the importance of the position and working for us.

Facilitated by Team Members

Career Opportunity Night is always facilitated by team members.

Depending on the position, it is usually facilitated by the team leader of that department. For example, when hiring a dental assistant, it's the clinical coordinator and a few dental assistants who'll facilitate the event.

Applicants get a first-hand look at the kind of people they're going to be working with. It's a great opportunity for our team to really shine.

It's also a great opportunity for applicants to really see what a bright future they can have with us.

Your team members are the best people to communicate how great it is because of their pride working with your team and the positions they hold within your practice.

As we often say, "People support what they help create." When the team members themselves handpick who's going to be the next team member, they invest personally in that person's success.

Hands-Off Approach

Team members actually run the entire event.

Dr. Meis: Do I do the sales pitch at the opportunity night?

Heather: I don't think they even invite you.

Dr. Meis: That's right. I don't even know they're going on.

We've been doing career opportunity nights now for several years. Dr. Meis did the first couple of events to model for the team what these events should look like. Over time, the team has taken over the event completely.

Each department is responsible for the further development of their own department and their own team.

In our office, whoever is directly responsible for the employee is the person who does the sales job and the hiring. If it doesn't work out, they're the ones who do the firing as well. That's our rule of thumb.

Observations During Career Opportunity Night

It is tremendously helpful and convenient to fill a room with applicants. It gives us the opportunity, in a single session, to see what they're all about.

To set up such an event, you should invite everyone. It doesn't matter how many potential applicants there are. Many times we've had our whole waiting room filled with potential applicants.

The team members' job is to observe everyone:

- What kind of attitude they come in with

- What they look like

- How they interact with other people

You can tell a tremendous amount about a person just by observing in a group like this.

Keep a look out for:

- **People who don't arrive on time.** This sets a bad tone. Maybe they got lost en route to the event, but you want someone who prepares and solves problems ahead of time. It is essential they arrive on time and present themselves well.

- **People who haven't said a word to anyone.** They're probably not much of a team player, or maybe they're too shy to be welcoming, warm and supportive with patients.

- **People with an inappropriate appearance for a dental practice.** We've had applicants with various visible angry-looking tattoos which certainly aren't very relaxing for patients.

- **People who attend the event dressed inappropriately.**

- **People who smell like smoke or alcohol or both.**

While observing the event, the team makes an *A* list and a *B* list. The *A* list candidates are those who interact well with other people, who look and act professionally, who came on time, and so on. It's an easy way for your team to narrow the field of candidates, and this should be done discreetly.

Everyone in attendance must feel just as likely to get the position as the person they're standing next to.

Offering Job Applications

After we've done our presentation selling potential applicants on the practice, we then ask those who are interested to fill out applications.

It's a non-intimidating and easy way for people to exit the process if they realize it's not the right fit. They can exit without having spent a lot of your time or theirs.

A very large percentage, although not 100%, of the attendees at career opportunity nights fill out an application. The most common reason that people don't fill out applications is because we don't have any part-time positions.

Debrief Immediately Afterwards

We always have a little debriefing session immediately following a career opportunity night. The team sorts the applications into an *A* pile and a *B* pile. The *A* pile are the candidates that they're most interested in and want to contact first for potential employment.

Holding a career opportunity night is a really effective and efficient way of narrowing down a large number of potential applicants for a job opening.

Sorting Through Your *A* Players

At our practice, we like to have mechanisms built in for sorting because conducting five to seven interviews is plenty.

We often have a short set of instructions for all career opportunity nights. When potential applicants are invited, they're asked to bring their resume and a cover letter or similar.

When only seven of the 15 potential applicants follow the specific instructions, for example, that brings our *A* pile down to seven. The rest are put back into the pipeline.

When that *A* pile is narrowed further, there's absolutely going to be at least three of those candidates you'll be torn between.

Interviewing

Preparing Managers for Interviews

When conducting interviews, the team member who'll manage that employee should do the interviews.

Here's a general guideline on who the interviewer should be in practices where there are:

- Five employees or less: the doctor

- Five to nine employees: the clinic administrator or office manager

- More than nine employees: the clinical manager or administrative manager, or both

- More than 15 employees: the practice manager who oversees both administrative and clinical departments

Have a set process for the interview. We prepare our managers in a handful of ways including explaining their responsibility to hire great people and how to look for attitude.

Have the conversation where *A* players hire other *A* players:

- *A* players are consistently improving and contribute to the success of the organization.

- *B* players don't drag a team down, but they don't positively improve the organization.

- *C* players are a bummer all the way around.

- *A* players will hire *A* players. *B* players will hire *B* and *C* players.

Put the responsibility on your managers to hire great people — the *A* players. If they don't feel like they have a great candidate, they're not ready to hire yet.

Educate Them on Attitude

Attitude is the most important criterion we use for hiring applicants. If they don't have a great attitude, they're not an *A* player, and it's time to move on to the next applicant.

Here's a general guideline to tell if an applicant has a great attitude:

- **Look for people who ask a lot of questions and challenge you.** They ask uncommon questions. They want to know a little bit more than the average person would regarding the practice or opportunities. Being challenged is almost always a very good sign.

- **They can develop a connection quickly.** We're given such a small opportunity to connect with patients, so you need people who can make a great impression in a short amount of time. People who are shy and timid often have difficulty in dental practices because they don't make connections easily and end up alienating patients.

- **They seem eager and motivated.**

- **They are inviting, outgoing, sociable and confident.**

Interview Questions

It's important to ask job candidates the right questions during an interview. Here are some quick tips to develop your interview questions:

- **Ask open-ended questions** (questions that should not yield a "yes" or "no" answer). The candidates' answers show how well they communicate and how creative they are. They can answer more in depth. They'll often times offer information you can't or don't feel comfortable asking for.

- **Think of four or five qualities a person with this job should have.** Craft questions asking them about their experience with those qualities. Some examples could include being part of a team, being a leader, problem solving or being in a mediator role. One question we often ask is, "Tell me about a time, it could in school, when you were in a leadership position and you had to make a decision."

- **Take the pressure off the candidates as much as you can.** Say, "I'm just looking for an example of when you did that. It can be anything. It can be something small."

- **Ask questions they won't have a pre-made response for.** We often have people say, "That's a really good question." They'll take time to actually think about it. They'll search their memory for a good example. When a candidate answers questions too quickly, we're a little concerned about the truth of the answer.

- **Score how well they respond.** Ask yourself these questions: Did they have an answer? Was it well-spoken and well thought out? If they respond, "I don't know, I've never been a leader" then, that's not who you're looking for.

- **Have a casual conversation.** Give them a chance to open up and talk about themselves professionally and personally. Put together a list of five questions that get candidates talking, so you can determine if they will be the right fit for your practice. Ask, "Where would you like to see yourself in five years? Do you have a family? An education?" Ask those types of questions.

- **Questions should be the same for every candidate.** There are legal reasons for this. It helps ensure you have a fair hiring process (which is an area where people commonly get into trouble with litigation). It's also easier for comparing candidates. By using the same questions, you're comparing apples to apples. It's easier to look objectively at their responses to determine who did the best job in that interview.

Heather:

We've learned a lot about interviewing over the years.

I look back at the beginning, and I think, "Wow, I feel sorry for those people. I didn't give them a fair chance to put themselves out there."

Back then, I just asked standard questions like, "What do you feel your biggest strength is?" Anyone can answer those, and they usually give you the answers they think you want to hear.

Good Indicators to Look For

There are three good indicators of candidates who will do well in a team-centered practice:

1. **They had a successful past in athletics (particularly team sports).** These candidates are better team members because to be successful in team sports, they had to learn the lessons, "It's not about me. It's about the team" and "It's about doing what I can do to make the team more effective." We ask questions about their experiences being on a successful team.

2. **Their parents own their own business.** These candidates understand money doesn't grow on trees. They've heard their parents talk about the struggles of owning their own business: dealing with employee

difficulties, the struggle to make payroll, and how challenging it is to run a business. Most of these candidates will also have worked in that business, usually starting at a young age, so they have a long history of work experience and a great work ethic, but that is not always the case.

3. **They worked as teenagers.** If they have a long history of being employed, it says a lot about their character because they probably always had to work, are used to working and likely enjoy it. They've had a lot of experience in the workforce, so they know what's expected of them.

When we find these indicators, we note it. We believe they're good indicators of people who will function well on our team.

Four Essential Qualities of Dental Success

There are four qualities that help a person be more successful in dentistry.

1. **Being empathetic.** They're able to get into the same emotional space as the patients. They connect with them wherever they are. Even though it's not taught in dental schools, it may be the single most important quality in dental success.

2. **Instant likability.** Dentistry is largely small talk with patients. You have a limited amount of time to connect and make an impact.

3. **Warm and welcoming.** Make sure that your people who are on the front line dealing with patients every day are warm and welcoming, especially those answering the phone.

Dr. Meis:

One of my friends recently became a patient at my practice. Apparently, his previous dentist never talked to him. The dentist would come in and look in his mouth, then instruct the assistant or hygienist, and he would leave.

My friend said he had more conversation in his first visit with us than he had in decades with this other dentist.

Being warm and welcoming is really important.

---

4. **Being attractive.** Attractive people have more success than unattractive people. Some people may take offense to that, but the research on it is clear (see Robert Cialdini's *Influence: The Psychology of Persuasion*). Candidates don't have to be models but they shouldn't be unattractive. Multiple facial piercings will be considered unattractive in my area, for example.

Candidates should be attractive in both personality and appearance. Patients have high expectations for the appearance of their health care provider.

Screening

After holding the career opportunity night, we usually have a pool of the best three to five applicants. We interview them and narrow the pool down to two or three candidates.
Then, we screen the final two or three candidates before making a final hiring decision. Note we aren't screening 15-20 people. Only the final few.

The Wonderlic Personnel Test (WPT)

Wonderlic calls it a test that measures a person's ability to learn. It appraises decision-making ability and practical skill sets such as reading comprehension and basic mathematics. It shows how well a person thinks on a broad spectrum.

Every dental job has complexity to it. No matter what position an employee holds, there is a lot to learn. Employees need to have the intelligence and learning ability necessary to work through these difficulties.

Kolbe A

We really enjoy Kolbe's results and people enjoy taking it. It is an assessment of the way a person likes to work. For example, some questions include:

- Are you someone who needs a great deal of facts before starting a project?

- Do you just jump right in and sort things out later?

- Do you like to build things with your hand?

This assessment shows how you're most comfortable approaching work.

The Kolbe A scores a person (from 1–9) in four categories:

- **Fact Finder.** If you score high in Fact Finder, you like to do lots of research and know everything before you get started. People who are high in fact finding can feel to others like they have paralysis by analysis. This may not be the case. They may just require more facts before starting than those with lower scores in this area.

- **Follow Through.** If given a new project, would you naturally be excited to work on that first, or would you finish existing projects before starting? If you're the latter, then you have a high Follow Through score.

- **Quick Start.** These are visionary people, big dreamers, but not always the best at following through or implementing.

- **Implementer.** These people depend on physical space and ability to operate manually.

There isn't a good score or a bad score. Each category has wonderful qualities and simply reflects who you are.

How We Use the Kolbe to Assess Candidates

As human beings, we tend to be drawn to people with similar characteristics, but the strongest teams come from diversity.

- If you had an entire team of dreamers, it'd be an extremely happy place where nothing got done.

There are Kolbe scores you would look for in certain positions.

- For example, with our financial controller, we want someone who pays attention to detail and has great follow through (rather than a visionary). We looked for someone with those specific characteristics.

Use Kolbe Scores to Improve Understanding Inside Your Team

No matter how great your team is, there'll occasionally be conflict. Often the conflict comes from a large difference in Kolbe's scores.

Our entire team has taken the Kolbe A. Everyone is aware of each other's score.

It has proved helpful in team building and creating teams for projects. We have a fuller understanding of each other. We have become much more responsible with how we approach each other and the expectations we have.

Dr. Meis:

Our financial controller is a very high fact finder. She and I are working together on a project right now that requires a lot of fact finding.

I don't have as much fact-finding skill, talent or desire as she does. It's not my primary mode. When she goes deep into facts, it goes beyond my attention span. I start to fade. I want to go on to the next thing. For this project, what she's doing is absolutely right.

That's why having that blend in diversity is really important. If we were all the same, we wouldn't be as effective.

The Internet as a Screening Tool

According to reports, 12% of employers use Google and other sites as their screening tools.

This may not be wise since there's a mix of accurate and inaccurate information on the Internet. However, if you want to do it, you should do it the right way.

If you Google one person, you need to Google every person. If you want to reject someone based on what you found online, you need to be upfront and inform potential candidates that you have checked or will be checking their information online.

Uncovering Information of a Personal Nature

You'll find out information on the Internet that you won't find on a job application or resume. You'll find information that should not be considered in the hiring process.

It's hard to say, "I did see they were of the Catholic faith on their Facebook page, but I did not consider that when hiring them." It's hard to prove you kept the neutral, job specific information in the forefront of your mind when you made the hiring decision. It's always easier not to do it than having to defend yourself after the fact.

You can get in trouble when you uncover protected characteristics (gender, race, religion, and so on) whether personally or by association. That information should not be and legally can't be considered when hiring an employee.

If you do use it, make sure you have a legitimate reason for why a person wasn't considered for the job, in case you need to defend yourself.

Drug Screening

Drug use is a safety concern. You don't want drugged out employees in charge of patient care.

This came to our attention when a group practice we work with found people were failing drug screenings even though they did well in all the other pre-employment interactions. Even high-level employees, like dentists, were failing drug tests.

Remember to be consistent: If you drug test one applicant, drug test them all. If you have a no tolerance policy, apply it evenhandedly. Even if one person is talented but fails a drug test, don't hire that person.

Background Checks

Do different levels of background checks based on the position you're trying to fill within the practice.

Have more in-depth background checks for positions that are making larger scale decisions such as associate doctors and financial controllers. Background checks are critical for anyone who is in charge of patient care or handling money.

Make an educated decision on whether that person should be a part of your team. You have the safety of your team members and your patients to consider.

Ordering Background Checks

Multiple companies provide background check services for a reasonable price. They provide a document for applicants to fill out, and turnaround is usually within a couple of days. Background checks can be as in-depth as you would like, and they can offer recommendations based on the position you're hiring for.

Request a Self-Disclosure or Authorization for a Background Check

Ask applicants for their permission to do a background check.

Often people will be upfront about their past (including actions they are not proud of). People will make confessions, "I've had speeding tickets. Does that count?"

A report doesn't always tell the entire story. Let them tell their side of the story.

Disclosure is Beneficial

Disclosure ahead of time is very beneficial, and it doesn't necessarily mean they won't be hired.

Like many practices, we've had people who didn't divulge their significant criminal histories.

The employment decision is easy when you can eliminate someone because of something significant in their background—particularly when it was undisclosed.

Dr. Meis:

When we were hiring a financial controller, one of the people who applied was very likable and sharp.

He had lots of really inventive ideas. When he left the interview, I thought he had a good chance of getting the job.

He was a former bank officer. The president of that bank was a friend of mine, so I asked about him. It turned out that he had falsified bank records and fraudulently given loans to friends. He was convicted in federal court, sentenced to prison and served a couple of years for the crime.

He should have been upfront. I would have felt totally different if he didn't wait until I found it out myself.

At the time, we used an informal background check, but after that experience we added a formalized background check.

Embezzlement

It's extremely common for dental practices to be ripped off through embezzlement.

Some form of embezzlement probably happens in every practice; for instance, employees not being 100% accurate on their time sheets or employees using work time for personal errands, Facebook or texting. These activities can be considered embezzlement if you carry the definition to the extreme.

People who have a history of theft usually have found some way to justify it in their head that it's acceptable. If they can get away with it once, they can do it again.

Protect your practice by having a background check on all job applicants.

Depth of Background Check

The depth of a background check should be equivalent to the position sought. An associate doctor, who is going to be writing prescriptions, should have a different type of background check than someone answering the phones at the front desk.

If you have multiple applicants for the same position, background and reference checks should be the same for everyone. You can't use a different standard for the same position.

Document the Screening

It's always good to inform applicants that you're going to be doing background checks and have them sign a simple consent form that includes the text "I understand all information will be verified; inaccurate information and purposefully misleading information will be grounds for termination." Often times, you find out after the test that someone wasn't completely truthful with the information they provided.

Negligence and Your Responsibility to Safety

Don't fail to protect your employees' and patients' safety.

We put team members in close proximity to people. Patients are sedated and in vulnerable positions. For the safety of your patients, team members and yourself, it's best to have some sort of due diligence.

Dr. Meis:

I know someone who owned an animal cop shop. They rounded up stray animals and enforced laws on pets.

This company had hired an employee without doing a background check. He turned out to be a serial rapist.

He used the badge and truck, which looked like a police vehicle, to commit crimes.

The Hiring Decision

You've got all the information. You've asked all the questions you wanted to. Next, it's decision time.

If you don't have a clear frontrunner, revisit which "seat on the bus" this person is going to fill.

- Look at the characteristics you're looking for in that position.

- Ask yourself which person fits that mold the best.

This decision is not always immediately clear in the beginning stages of hiring. Over time, it'll get easier. You'll become more intuitive and more confident in your decisions.

Dr. Meis:

We once had two applicants who were virtually identical: same Kolbe scores, both were good matches, highly intelligent and nice people, and both had certification we were looking for.

When you have two great applicants, you can't go wrong. That's really a great place to be.

Making an Employment Offer

Our job offer is always congratulatory: "We've decided we'd love to have you join our team."

We always present an employment as a great celebration — because it is. It's the start of a huge opportunity for them and for us.

Training

Their First Day

The biggest challenge in hiring and the part that scares many people is what happens after you've got them in the door and what comes next. We've learned a few things over the years.

Start Their First Day on the Job Later in the Week

We used to start new hires on a Monday because it was the beginning of the week—but an entire week right away can be overwhelming.

Now, we start new hires on Wednesday or Thursday. They work a day or two and then have the weekend. It starts everything on a good note. They think, "Oh, that was great." Then, we start full force the next week.

Acclimate Them to the Practice on their First Day

Establish best practices for when you're acclimatizing new hires on their first day on the job:

- Introduce them to everyone at the practice

- Inform them where things are kept

- Fill out necessary paperwork

- Teach them how to clock-in and clock-out

There are federal forms that are essential and mandatory. Have a system that requires new hires to bring all the relevant documentation that are federally mandated, including social security card and driver's license, on their first day of work.

At your practice, absolutely ensure that best practices are established for collecting a new hire's information within the first three days, otherwise you'll end up in a quandary; you don't want to be saying, "We have to track them down. We never got that." or "Oh gosh! Thirty days have gone by and we've forgotten to verify their documentation."

The Training Process

After the new hire's first day, we dive in fairly quickly from there with a set of training expectations.

Is Training an Event or Is It a Process?

People often think of training as an event: "You're new. You're trained. There you go." That's not the case. It really is more of a process.

3-3-3 System

At one time, our practice had a more traditional training system. We put new employees with a person who was in charge of teaching them everything. The responsibility was more than on the trainee. It was draining for the trainer and not as motivating for the trainee.

We learned a much better system from Stonehaven Dental called the 3-3-3.

With this system, you set your expectations for new employees to reach a set of goals within 3 days, 3 weeks and 3 months. For example, we tell new employees, "You need to know these five tasks within 3 days, these 10 within 3 weeks and these 25 within 3 months." These aren't insurmountable tasks. The bar is relatively low.

- The 3-day tasks are no-brainers.

- The 3-weeks tasks are a little more in-depth.

- At 3 months, new employees have to be independent in their jobs.

New employees are given the resources necessary to accomplish everything, including a mentor if they need help along the way. It's their responsibility to make sure they accomplish these goals.

People are able to learn at their own pace, but the deadlines make sure it doesn't any take longer than it needs to.

Using this system takes much of the effort of training off the mentor and puts it on the trainee.

Assessing New Employees with the 3-3-3 System

Just because you hired new employees, doesn't mean you have to live with them forever.

By giving new employees the responsibility to accomplish all the tasks on their 3-3-3 list, you can quickly figure out if they aren't going to make it.

- Remember, we want employees who get it, want it, and can do it. They should come with batteries included. They shouldn't require much effort and energy from other people to get them pumped up and to get them through.

- If they don't work through the 3-3-3 or don't do it well, we know it won't work.

Employees Benefit from the 3-3-3 System

New employees appreciate guidelines and deadlines.

Usually by day two, employees are already moving on to the 3-week criteria. That makes them feel really good. It allows them to move along at a pace that's comfortable for them as well. It gives them some early wins to increase their confidence.

All of us perform better when we're coming from a place of confidence. This is one way to get new employees off on the right foot.

It adds a level of excitement because new employees, especially dental assistants, can be very eager to get started:

- Before the 3-3-3, they always asked, "How soon am I going to be doing that?" The 3-3-3 system lays everything out.

- They understand that they aren't just going to be standing around watching for an excessive amount of time.

- They get excited to look ahead and see they are going to be doing a certain task in no time at all.

Creating the 3-3-3 for Each Position

We have a 3-3-3 process for each employee type: one for dental assistants, one for dental hygienists, one for the administrative staff, and so on.

In creating the 3-3-3 roadmap, we sat down with team leaders and listed our expectations of each position. Then, we drew a timeline:

- **3 Days.** There are things that make sense to know right away. These are the no-brainers you can easily accomplish.

- **3 Weeks.** These are the essential things to know.

- **3 Months.** These are things that are the most difficult or time-intensive.

We then took it back to the teams in different departments and asked, "What should the 3-3-3 be?" They started filling it with their contributions.

Team Involvement in the 3-3-3

We want everyone we hire to be a success. We make sure we do everything we can to help them develop into great employees and positive additions to the teams. We want them to be able to make our patient service even better.

By blending our ideas with our team's ideas, we came up with something everyone really bought into. Since they were a part of creating it, they're great at carrying through with it as trainers and mentors. They understand what the system is.

They understand their roles. They're absolutely committed and understand how they can help someone be a success.

Team members sometimes have higher expectations for themselves and their teammates than we do. They'll say flat out, "Absolutely, you should know that in three weeks. It's not that difficult. You need to know that." They raise the bar for each other.

Employees Who Do Not Complete the 3-3-3

If something goes wrong at the beginning, it's probably going to continue to unravel.

One shared characteristic in elite practices is that when something isn't working, they change it quickly. They don't drag things out, trying to decide "Will this work? Won't this work?"

The 3-3-3 is pretty clear. If they aren't able to accomplish the tasks, they aren't a good fit for the practice. We then make decisions quickly for the employees' benefit and for ours.

It's horrible to be stuck in a job that's not right for you, or one that you don't enjoy or aren't good at. That's really a bad place to be in life. When we have employees who are there, we respectfully help them move on to a different future.

You're not doing them any favor by holding onto them. It deflates everyone else. It's especially deflating for the one who's performing poorly.

Personal Development Interview

A Personal Development Interview (PDI) is a key part of each employee's development.

First, Break All the Rules is a business book by Curt Coffman that explores the common qualities of highly successful companies. One shared trait the author found was having great employee interactions. Employees felt someone in the company was interested in their development. This was an inspiration for the PDIs.

What is a PDI?

- Managers meet with each employee who reports to them.

- Meetings are held weekly or biweekly, depending on their experience and tenure.

- The idea is to develop objectives for each one of your employees to make them an even more valuable part of the team.

- Once objectives are determined, simply ask questions during the meetings that'll lead the employee to fulfill their objectives.

PDIs, as a strategic management system, are effective because they are consistent.

Occasionally, people have an "Ah-ha!" moment and make radical and sudden changes. That doesn't happen often. Change usually happens much slower. The PDI system is setup to help people have those "Ah-ha!" moments that change behaviors quickly, but if that doesn't happen, it allows them to have that change over time.

- Each team member knows that they are going to meet with you every week.

- You'd always ask them how they have improved. When team members know they're going to be held accountable, it's easy for them to start adhering to objectives.

- Team members clearly understand what is important. Otherwise, you won't be repeatedly asking them the same question.

- It's a comfortable way to discuss what they're doing well and what they're not doing so well. When they struggle with something, it becomes a new objective.

Employees appreciate that there's time set aside that you've committed to their success. If you try to skip a PDI, team members will chase you down and remind you. It's that valuable to them.

Motivational and Non-Disciplinary

PDIs are motivational meetings. If you have a performance issue, don't use PDIs to begin the discussion. If you have to reprimand someone, that's a separate meeting.

You may add an interview question about an issue they need to work on, but don't make PDIs downers. PDIs are never downers. No one will want to show up for 30-minute lectures every week. You have to keep it motivating.

PDIs should always make people feel more valuable, confident and that they are making progress (when they are) on their path of personal development.

Make sure you don't send contradictory messages at PDIs. Don't tell them everything's fantastic if it isn't, but do maintain a motivating environment.

If you had a disciplinary conversation previously about arriving on time, for instance, you can certainly follow up in your PDI and say, "I see you were on time four of the five days last week. Tell me how you made that change." Reward them for progress. We always say, "Progress, not perfection." The more you reward their progress, the quicker they get to where you want them to be.

This is the opposite of the typical carrot-and-stick management style many dentists were taught. The carrot for people with the PDI system is their own personal development, and there is no stick. They're not going to lose their job. There's no yelling.

Employees want what's good for them and what's good for the practice. Help them get there and make them feel confident they can do it. Many employees feel we have expectations beyond what is possible. With the PDI system, we help them understand it's possible and that we're going to help them to get there.

Objections to the PDI

Cutting into production is the biggest concern administrators and owners have with starting PDIs.

Abraham Lincoln said, "If I was given six hours to chop down a tree, I'd spend the first five hours sharpening my axe." Sharpening an axe feels non-productive but, in reality, it makes you more productive.

PDIs are the best way we've found to do that. It makes you more productive because it gets team members to focus on a bigger future for the practice and themselves.

Since we started doing PDIs several years ago, our need for disciplinary conversations has shrunk. This is because we took the time to develop people and clarify our expectations.

PDI Questions

Some questions are universal. Most are unique to each employee. They're developed specifically to help that employee get to the next level.

Here is how the typical interview goes:

- One question we ask everyone is, "What have you done to create a motivating environment in the office?"

- If someone is having difficulty creating a motivating environment, we would ask, "What did you do this week to create a motivating environment?"

- Team members will search for something. If they haven't done anything, they'll go silent.

- Leave them in that uncomfortable spot. Don't say anything. Just ask the question and wait for them to come up with a response.

- They may not have a response for the first couple of weeks. They just sit there in that uncomfortableness and say, "I really haven't done anything to create a motivating environment." They have to admit it.

- In our system, we don't make a big deal if they haven't done anything. We just say, "Well, I know you've been busy and things have been tough, but what could you do during the next week to create a motivating environment?"

- Be very quiet. Don't give them ideas. Just let them think about it. Let there be an uncomfortable silence.

By doing this over and over again with a recurring topic, people will get it over time, if they don't have an eureka moment.

PDIs are very clear-cut. Team members should get it whether they want to do it or can do it. If they aren't getting it, it's an indicator you have someone that either can't do it or won't do it.

Remember, you're trying to weed out poor performers. Give employees every chance to develop. If they still aren't developing, if they just can't get it or don't want it, then you move them out of your practice and make room for someone who will.

Learning Each Team Member's Motivation

It's beneficial to use that time to learn more about each team member.

What brings them to work every day?

What do they want to accomplish for themselves as a person?

Heather:

One of our associate doctors loves Nebraska football. He would love to spend the entire PDI talking about Nebraska football. As a practice, we'd like him to do more same-day dentistry.

I'll often ask, "What did you do last week to make yourself more available for same-day treatment?"

He'll then do some hemming and hawing.

Things don't happen overnight, but the more we talked about it, the more he naturally morphed into being able to provide same-day dentistry.

I then made a joke about it and said, "One more crown and you're that much closer to season tickets."
Those little things provide a nice atmosphere.

I try to make team members realize that "I want you to be just as successful as I want the practice to be, and together we can make both of those things happen."

Figure out what they are hoping to accomplish and relate the two together.

Correlate their personal objectives with the goals of the practice. Connect their accomplishment and development at work with their own personal desires.

For instance, all our employees have the opportunity to earn more money. If we have a person who wants a certain possession, we have opportunities that can help them fund it. We can relate how their behavior in the practice can help them get what they want. The same applies to employees with more mission-oriented goals.

We also have people who are motivated by creating a great team environment. Knowing that, you then ask questions that help them on that pathway of getting better at creating one.

Check in With Your Employees in Some Way

We encourage everyone to set up some form of consistent check-in with your team members. Set aside time even if it feels like it's cutting into productivity. It makes a huge difference. You'll be amazed at the results you get.

Legal Issues

We're not giving any legal advice here; what we're giving is information about some of the legal aspects of hiring, developing and firing employees.

We aim to bring awareness to potential legal hazards. Laws vary from state to state. Consult an expert party before making any legal decisions.

Consistency

The biggest problem in hiring and firing is being inconsistent. When everyone isn't treated the same, you can get into serious trouble whether it's applicants, employees or those being fired.

A lack of consistency leaves you at risk for having the problem of unfair labor practices.

Usually, it's not that people want to be unfair. They just don't have a systematic way of approaching it. They do it one way one day, then another way the next day.

Regardless of intent, this can be misinterpreted as unfair or giving advantage to one or the other.

It's always better to have done it right the first time rather than trying to go back and explain, "Even though it doesn't look right, trust us. We're fair."

Consistency in Gathering the Information

If you do or don't collect resumes, be consistent. If you call two or three references listed on person A's resume or application, call two out of the three listed on person B. Just make sure that every time the same process is being followed.

What applies for one position would apply for all so long as each applicant is treated the same way.

Common Lawsuits

These kinds of lawsuits are common. Attorneys see them as easy money. All they have to do is allege unfair labor practices, and you have to prove that your labor practices aren't unfair. That's difficult and expensive to do. Many practices just settle, and since they settle, it's easy money.

Applicant Screening

Remember, in applicant screening, we treated everyone the same. We had everyone come in to the practice, and we had the same process for everyone at the career opportunity night. Everyone had the opportunity to fill out an application, then we made an A pile and a B pile based upon written criteria.

The criteria that we use at the practice is simple, and it is written down:
- The applicant showed up on time.

- The applicant was dressed appropriately.

- They had no visible piercings and tattoos.

- They did not smell like smoke.

- They had positive interaction with other people.

Generating Interest in a Position

When generating a pool of interest into your practice, have a consistent process however you do it, so you know everyone's being treated fairly.

Careful in Conversation

Be careful as seemingly harmless conversation can often take you to areas that shouldn't be discussed.

Reviewing Resumes

When reviewing resumes, try to put up blinders. Ignore facts that are of a personal nature and aren't job-specific. Get thoughts like these out of your mind: "Oh, that person worked at McDonald's," or "Oh, they graduated high school in 19xx."

Whether we address our personal biases or not, do what you can to avoid interactions with details of a personal nature.

Cover up the objective portion or anything that will give any personal information—someone's name (you can tell a lot by their name) or where they lived—just look at job-specific information.

Begin by sorting out your *A* pile and your *B* pile based on job-specific type of criteria.

Create a Checklist

Focus on the key characteristics of the position, such as supervisory experience. Look at a resume: Does the applicant have such experience? It doesn't matter where they learned those skills (even if it came from McDonald's). Are those characteristics shown in the applicant's resume?

Be sure you're focusing on exactly what it is that you have set out as being the most relevant and important experience.

For example, if you're hiring a hygienist to give local anesthesia and an applicant isn't certified, you can reject their resume for that reason. If another applicant is certified, put that resume in the *A* pile. Then, look at the other characteristics or experiences you're looking for to sort through that *A* pile.

Have exactly what you're looking for written down, and then stick to it. Use the neutral criterion, "Does that person have that?"

Use Job Applications

If you don't screen resumes, job applications are an absolute necessity. If you do screen resumes, still have a job application. It's a great way to ensure that the exact same information is being requested from every applicant.

Unacceptable Criteria

You can't use certain criteria for hiring or not hiring.

Protected classes include religion, age and gender. The list varies from state to state, and many classes that you wouldn't even think are protected, in fact, are protected. Be clear on what is unacceptable in your state.

Clear Expectations

Job Descriptions

Be sure employees understand exactly what the duties and responsibilities are associated with the position which they've been hired for.

Sometimes, people apply and aren't a good fit for one position but will be well-suited for another position. If this happens, let them know the position they're being hired for. Job descriptions are essential.

Hiring in Writing

Once you've found a candidate you think is a good fit, have clearly defined terms of what your relationship's going to be. Know the terms of employment.

Some people may hire an associate dentist based on a contract as compared to at will. There are different circumstances for each.

- **At Will.** The employee can be let go for any type of violation. Most states fall in the at-will category these days unless you set forth a contract for employment. You can hire and fire anyone for any legal reasons at any given time. There's not a definite term to the employment relationship. There isn't a specific list of situations that'll lend themselves to termination. The employee can leave at any time; the employer can terminate at any time.

- **Contract.** The obligations of the employer and the employee are specifically set forth in the contract such as "We're hiring you on *x* term for *x* number of years or for an undetermined amount of time, and the only ways that we can end this employment relationship are X, Y and Z." The relationship can only end under the terms set forth in the contract. Contract employees are confined to the terms of the contract.

Note: Just because they have a contract doesn't mean they aren't an at-will-employee because you can state it in the contract that they are an at will employee. Most associate doctors are also at will employees according to their contracts.

If you have an at will employee, often there is some sort of document that sums up the employment relationship. Be very clear in stating that despite the certain terms that accompany the relationship, it remains at will and just causes are not needed for termination.

Sign on the Dotted Line

Have employees sign a fact sheet stating they understand the terms of employment—the employment relationship, hours, pay, vacation, benefits, and so on. Make them acknowledge that they're fully aware of what they're getting into.

Hours, Pay and Vacation

Always be upfront. Many practices have work hours that aren't 9–5. People often say they're available for certain hours, but when they get into it, they say "I didn't really think you'd make me work every Friday," and reasons like that. So, set expectations for hours and the variation in hours. If it's not going to be a set schedule, lay that out upfront.

Broken promises create negative feelings. State what the pay scale is and what the starting wage is. Ensure there are no promises you can't meet or don't intend to meet.

Shifting Standards Create Disgruntled Employees

Shifting standards cause problems to occur quickly. Here's an example:

Management states they have a starter wage and after x number of weeks or months, they'll bump an employee up.
This causes the employee to have that expectation (because that was the expectation given to them).

But for whatever reason, a change of mind, a whim or poor performance, the employee doesn't get the pay bump.

Because of the expectation, the employee feels entitled to it. Now, they feel they've been treated unfairly.

If you're promising a bump up, then regardless of how things go, they have an expectation you failed to live up to. It's the perfect way to have an employee start off a little disillusioned and quickly turn to a disgruntled employee.

If you do have a bump up, but you aren't consistently applying it on the same level or time frame that can be seen as inconsistency and unfair treatment.

Add Flexibility into the Job Description

As employers, we would love to have the responsibilities and duties listed as: "Anything that needs to be done. Anything I tell you to do."

We want flexibility. If you have a need in another area, you can move people around, so the needs of the practice and patients are taken care of.

We achieve this by hiring people for a specific job with a specific set of responsibilities and duties, but we also include a paragraph that coveys, "We're in a business of serving patients, and you may be used in a capacity other than this based on your talent."

Avoid creating a situation where there's no latitude for someone (outside of defined characteristics that are listed in the job description).

However, a clearly defined job description can be a good starting point when it comes to disciplining and setting expectations.

It's a nightmare to have the practice need something done but employees say, "It's not in my job description."

In 25 years of practice, I've never had anyone say that. However, in consulting with other practices, it does happen. That's a good indicator of someone who doesn't have the attitude you want in your practice.

Employee Handbook

There are many legal concerns, and it may seem like a lot to bite off at once. If you don't have a good employee handbook, create one because that's the first place to start.

Get a good set of eyes to review it. If you do have one, make sure it's up-to-date and offers the protection you think you need. We use HR Consultants at our practice. They're not attorneys, but they can give you good advice. They often have a handbook process for creating good and legal employee handbooks.

An employee handbook is always good to have because all employees will have the same information.

Management has a resource to consult with, so it can be applied in a consistent manner.

It sets the same expectation for everyone and avoids the appearance of any bit of favoritism. The policies are right there for everyone.

Have new employees sign and acknowledge they received an employee handbook. In addition, have them acknowledge they have read and understand the policies contained within it.

Some employee handbooks tend to be a little too detailed. You never want to forfeit the at will relationship by having any statements that give the employee the assurance of job security or lead them to believe there's only certain circumstances that'll lead to termination.

We highly recommend getting professional help. You can get caught in a bad spot if you don't have this done properly. Review your employee handbook on an annual basis. Do this even if you feel like your handbook's been around for a long time, and it has always served you well. Things change over time. Make sure it's keeping up.

Look for words like 'may' or 'should' as opposed to 'shall' or 'must.'

For example, "must use the vacation prior to taking a maternity leave" versus "may use the vacation prior to taking a maternity leave." If person A is taking maternity leave and doesn't use her vacation but person B is told they need to use her vacation prior to maternity leave, it's a huge discrepancy and treatment of people.

Those kinds of phrases leave for a little bit of waffling in management situations. There may be loopholes for differential treatment of employees who are very similarly situated.

Disciplinary Process

Documenting Training Sessions

Often when you get to the disciplinary stage of employment, employees will shift the blame.

"Well, I didn't know I had to do that," or "No one told me that was part of my job," or "I wasn't trained in that area."

A lot of time and energy goes into training and bringing employees up to speed and maintaining performance.

It's a good habit, especially in group training sessions, to pass around an attendance list or an acknowledgment form that states "I was present at this training session."

So, if you do end up in a disciplinary situation where you have someone who has excuses but aren't meeting expectations, you have documentation that you have provided them adequate training. It shifts the burden back to employees who may not be pulling their weight.

Difficult and Disciplinary Conversations

When you have an employee who isn't performing like you think they should, the intention of these conversations is to get the employee on track and to help them perform at a level that's acceptable. These conversations are for the employee's benefit.

Be Very Direct and Totally Honest

Most people who go into dentistry have a very kind and nurturing side. This is part of what attracted us to this occupation. We're healers, and we want people to feel good. It may be contrary to your nature but you have to be brutally honest and do it in a kind way.

Many people think, "If I'm nice, it will make things a little bit easier. I'll try to get my point across, then hopefully things will improve, and there won't be so much tension in our day-to-day interaction."

When you bring something to someone's attention, there's no need to be negative or rude. Just give an honest assessment of what's taking place and what needs to be changed.

You're blocking someone's progress if you don't give them honest feedback. You're doing them a disservice.

It becomes difficult to resolve the problem if you haven't set out expectations and told them what the problem is or how deep it runs. You're not giving a clear indication of what you expect and a clear path for moving forward.

If there is a specific rule or policy violation, point it out in the employee handbook and direct them to review it.

Establish explicitly "You're being warned" or "You're being disciplined." Many mangers think, "I warned them," but depending on how straightforward you are, the employee may not perceive that as a warning.

Disciplinary Action Should be Done Face-to-Face and in Private

Disciplinary action shouldn't happen in a group environment.

Some managers try to address issues anonymously in a group. Even if it feels obvious who you're talking about, it may not be clear to them.

There is no way around it. You have to interact directly and specifically with the employee.

Stay Focused

- Avoid being overly detailed.

- Keep things extremely job-specific.

- Discuss nothing personal (unless the issue is of a personal nature, like they showed up for work smelling of alcohol).

Document Disciplinary Conversations

It's difficult to prove that an employee was warned if you have no documentation of it. Having a document that'll serve as as evidence is important.

Write a brief summary of what happened, including the reason for the discipline, the policy violation if there is one, and the date. Both the employee and manager should sign it.

If you have an employee who refuses to sign it, which happens more often than you'd think, note that they refused to sign it but that you did have the conversation.

The Disciplinary Process

Here is the disciplinary process we use in our practice:

1. We have a face-to-face conversation.

2. We sit down and have a written conversation if the performance doesn't improve.

3. We do a very serious written warning that conveys, "If this does not improve, you'll lose your job." Of course, it's not written in those words, but we make sure that the message is clear.

Exceptions to the Process

Obviously, the disciplinary process depends upon the seriousness of the matter.

If there's a theft involved or a matter of personal safety, don't follow these steps. Terminate employment immediately. The full disciplinary process is used when employees simply aren't performing up to standards.

Never promise there is going to be a certain set of actions before termination can occur. If there's something serious, like a theft, you shouldn't have to give that person a verbal warning.

Nothing in your employee handbook should say, "You'll be given a verbal warning before you're even terminated," or anything like that. You definitely want latitude in how you approach serious situations.

Personnel File

Everyone should have a personnel file. Documentation of disciplinary actions should be housed in their personnel file. All employees' disciplinary reports should be held together in the same filing system.

Termination

When it's time to terminate an employee, have documentation supporting how you arrived at this point. Keep it short and sweet and send them on their way.

- Tell them the reason they're being terminated but don't go into details.

- You don't have to give them time to explain and have it turn into an argument.

- Just say, "Here's the reason; you were warned about this."

Response to Termination

If you haven't walked the employee up to the point of termination, it often takes them completely by surprise.

Termination should never come as a surprise.

- They may leave the building quietly, but you're going to hear from them later.

- They're caught off guard, so they'll feel the punishment doesn't fit the crime.

I can't tell you how many times former team members in other practices have told me they were stunned.

They got fired, and they didn't see it coming. They didn't know that they weren't performing up to standards.

They're hurt. Hurt people often react angrily. Often, that first angry activity is to call an employment lawyer to see if there's anything that "can be done about this."

Breaking the News to the Rest of the Team

Other team members are going to wonder what happened.

Don't go into details. From a legal standpoint, this can lead to defamation, suits, slander, and so on.

It also causes unrest within the team to provide too many details. They're just not necessary.

Just say, for example, "Effective today, Susie is no longer employed here. We will have to come up with a plan to cover the phones in her absence." That's all that needs to be said.

Be Prepared for Worst Case Scenarios

You need to make sure the safety of your remaining employees is ensured.

Make sure the person's key has been returned, access to the building has been limited and other things of that nature.

If the employee being terminated reacts in a way that the police need to be involved, do whatever it takes to make sure your team is safe.

Always have two people in on this conversation with the employee, so it's not a one person's word against another. Have the person pack their stuff and leave immediately.

Have someone there when they're packing and walking them out. Make sure nothing confidential leaves the building. You hate to think about things like this, but it happens all the time.

Hiring Hygienists

Compensation Models for Hygiene

One of the things you should make clear before hiring hygienists is the compensation model. You need to know what you're going to offer.

It is critical that you have some type of production-based compensation in place. Hourly pay breeds laziness in many employees, especially providers.

Many doctors experience frustration with hygiene and hygiene productivity because their compensation structure has never been setup as a win-win.

Creating a Win-Win for Everyone

Many hygiene providers are wary of production-based compensation because a lot is outside of their control.

The essential structure of an effective compensation model should have:

- **A security net so they don't panic.** Most hygienists are reluctant to go full commission even though that's how they can get the maximum amount of compensation in a well-run practice.

- **More compensation on higher production days.** When hygienists work hard and do well with promoting same-day, preventive services or periodontal services, they know there's something in it for them at the end of the day. This creates a more productive employee from the beginning.

The Formula

Here's a simple formula that works best with hygienists who don't have an assistant.

The accepted principle is that hygienists should produce about three times what they earn.

- **The Daily Base.** Set the daily base at three times what the hygienist is being paid.

- **Additional Compensation.** Anything they produce above that number, compensate them an additional 10% or 15%. This varies based on the incentives you have in place: If they're part of a team bonus, it may only be 10%; if it's their only incentive, offer a higher percentage.

To illustrate, if they're currently making $300 a day, their daily base is $900. When they produce above $900, they receive an additional percentage.

It's the easiest model in a transition period. Nothing has to change. The salary stays the same, but if they produce three times what they're paid, there's something extra in it for them at the end of that day.

The Formula for Hygienists with an Assistant

If the hygienist has an assistant, adjust these numbers.

Add your hygienist to your assistant's salary, and multiply by three. That's a more ideal base in typical situations.

If they already average $1,500 a day with an assistant, it doesn't make sense to have the daily rate start at $1,000.

If they already average a decent production, start the base at $1,400 because if they consistently produce above their average, there's still something additional in it for them.

Underlying Principles in the Formula

There are different formulas based on whether you're assisted or non-assisted, but the general principle is the same.

Decide on a base that makes sense from a financial standpoint but don't set the base too high.

Remember, you're not giving them 100% of what they produce above that base. It's only 10% or 15%. There's still plenty of profitability left for the practice, even after that additional percentage is paid. Every additional dollar of production, the overhead on that dollar decreases as you go.

If you set the base too high, it's demoralizing. The hygiene team will look at it and say, "We're never going to hit that."

Avoid the Knee-Jerk Reactions—Don't Nickel and Dime

"My hygienist is already making plenty of money. I don't want to pay them anymore" is a common knee-jerk reaction.

Sometimes we focus on the wrong number. When you actually run the numbers, often even though you're writing out an additional amount to your hygienist, the practice is often way farther ahead than where it would have been if production had not increased. The more they take home, the more the doctor takes home.

The more production they do, the more profit there is in the practice in general. It's incentive for the hygiene team to be productive. When they are more productive, everyone wins.

When practices go from an hourly wage to production-based compensation, the productivity, energy level and happiness of employees jump. That means more patients are being taken care of in a better way.

Even after implementation of the compensation model, some doctors still drag their feet.

- Take the leap. Don't nickel and dime. Don't worry.

- Production jumps significantly once these changes are made. It's often 30%–40% overnight.

- Production will increase dramatically if this was the only change you made and nothing else was implemented.

Hygiene Delivery Model

Decide your delivery model before you hire anyone.

Clarify your delivery model to understand hiring needs:

- You may not need to hire a replacement even if you're one person down.

- You may need to try an assisted model. If it works, you may not need to hire a replacement, but you may need to hire a qualified hygiene assistant instead.

Be able to describe your model very simply and carefully so that potential hygienists understand what you're doing:

- Words like "assisted" and "accelerated" are often thrown around, but they aren't very clearly and universally defined. For example, some people think of an accelerated model as assisted hygiene even though there are significant differences.

- Hygienists' opinions of these methods vary because their application varies greatly.

Attracting the Right Candidates

Be Clear About What You're Looking For

You want someone who has these traits:

- Patient-focused

- A team player
- Energetic and enthusiastic
- Thrive under an incentive program
- Good at talking to people
- A winning attitude
- Flourish in a team environment

Hire for Personality

We believe you should hire for personality. You can teach the rest of the necessary skills. Look more for personality than the skill sets on the resume.

Detecting Personality

Personality is hard to detect just by looking at a resume or sometimes even on the phone.

Use a Temp Agency

We all have hygienists that need days off. Have temps come in and replace them when it's time to hire someone; find those people who filled in and did an excellent job—the ones whom everyone liked and got along with.

Approach Your Staff

Often, team members have friends, associates or school classmates who may be looking for a hygienist position. Personal recommendations from trusted people should carry a certain weight.

Use Careful Wording in Your Ads

The words you're using in the ad help weed out many potential applicants who may not fit what you're looking for.

Using words in the ad such as "highly motivated," "patient-focused," "team player," and so on are going to weed out those who just want the nine-to-five paycheck. If you're not highly motivated, what are the odds you're going to respond to an ad that advertises "highly motivated."

It's not a bad idea to mention in the ad or tell applicants initially that it's a production-based compensation structure. If they're not interested in functioning under that structure, chances are they're not highly motivated.

Mention your delivery method: "You're going to be working hand-in-hand with a highly trained assistant who'll make your job easier once you're providing services for our patients." Some hygienists may not want to use that delivery model.

That helps everyone to be very clear on what's expected.

Interview Questions for Providers

These questions determine the winning attitude and identify top hygienists.

- **Ask what their production averages are.** If they know that number off the top of their head, it's a solid indicator of a good prospect. They're on top of what they personally can provide. Note: If they don't know their numbers, it doesn't mean they're not a good prospect. It's either positive or neutral.

- **Ask about their familiarity with current techniques.** Are they trained and have they used a laser (if it is permissible in your state)? Are they familiar with the software you're using? And so on. These are going to help you know how much training needs to happen.

- **Ask about their continuing education in recent years and who it was with.** This shows the philosophies they've been trained with, and it helps you ascertain their personality as well.

- **Ask why they left their last office or looking for new work.** This can give you a glimpse into their personality and help you avoid some trouble down the road.

Dr. Meis:

One of the key things in highly functioning practices is the ability for the hygienist to be a team player.

One of my friends jokes about the hygienist in their offices. He calls them "High-genists," meaning they think they're higher than everyone else.

It's a mindset that is fading away, thankfully. Having people who see themselves as one more cog in the machine is key.

- **Ask what they have done in their past and what they are willing to do for you in the future.**

  - Are you willing to give injections on behalf of the doctor?" (assuming that it's legal in your state)

  - "Are you comfortable taking impressions?"

  - "How long has it been since you placed a sealant? Are you comfortable placing sealants?" We've worked with hygienists who haven't placed a sealant in 20 years. Can they learn how to do it again? Are they willing to? Some are. Some aren't.

  - "Are you willing to donate your time toward charitable efforts?"

  - "Are you willing to donate your time to a Dentistry with a Heart event?"

Are They Demanding or Accommodating?

Do they make demands or do they ask what you want?

Sometimes, a hygienist will come in and say, "If I'm going to work here, I have to have this and this." That's an indicator that you don't have the right fit.

The "Whatever It Takes" Exercise

This seems random, but it is a tried and true tactic.

On the way to the interview location, whether it's in the doctor's office or wherever it may be, have a trash can in view. Have a piece of paper crumpled up in a ball on the floor next to the trashcan.

If the person stops, picks it up and throws it away, it tells you a lot about their personality, that:

- They're willing to do whatever it takes.
- They take the initiative to fix it a problem when they see one.
- They don't have to be asked.
- They're motivated.
- They pay attention to detail.

There's a lot you can tell from that simple exercise.

Team Member Involvement

Many times the doctor is the only one involved in the hiring process, but the opinions of your team matter, especially with a provider.

During the hiring process, include other hygienists in the practice and the hygiene assistants they're going to be working with directly.

They often have a better insight into the team player quality than you will. They get a feel for the person much faster than a doctor will.

Applicants usually show the doctor a little different side of themselves than they show the staff; it's just a part of human nature. By involving your team, you'll get more knowledge because your team will see things you're blind to.

Working Interviews

With many employees, a working interview isn't a good idea. With a hygienist, it's almost critical to have one.

When it comes to a provider, you need to have at least a few days where you can test them out, and they can test you out before there's an offer or a permanent contract.

You don't have to call it a working interview. You can pay them temporary wages, but they need to come in and work a couple of days.

There are things you can't tell from their resume or the job interview. For example, you need to see how timely they are and how well they work with your team members.

See How Hygienists are With Patients

You need to see how they are with patients—how they talk to patients, how they treat patients and how patients respond to them.

Patient feedback should be a critical component of the hiring process. Take surveys of the patients after they're finished.

It's even a wise strategy to have a couple of ringers as their patients. Ringers are people who'll be brutally honest with you about their treatment. They need to tell you if it was painful.

A hygienist often has your patient's undivided attention for 30 to 60 minutes. Having a hygiene provider that's not a good fit can cause some damage to the practice. If you've got someone who's causing your patients a lot of discomfort or pain, patients will start leaving in droves.

Hygienists Need to See If It is the Right Fit for Them

They'll see if your delivery model suits them. It may not.

The hygienist may want an assisted model, for example. If they expect an assistant to help them to type data, it's something you both need to know from the beginning.

Training

A New Hygienist's Traditional First Day

Hygienists are often only told on their first day, "Here's your instruments. Here's the lab. Here's your stuff. Ready? Go."

That's challenging because although a lot is the same, they still need training regarding your practice. For example, they need to understand what you expect of them and your philosophy.

Head Start on Training

Our online courses are a valuable training resource for new hygienists. We recommend you have the new hire watch at least the first four sessions on preventive services before their first day.

It helps new hygienists get an idea of their role as a preventive therapist from the very beginning. It shows where we'd like them to start and how we try to serve our patients.

They see that patients should have every opportunity presented to them that would benefit them.

The very first day that they start, they're offering fluoride. They're talking with patients about sealants, desensitizing possibilities and other things like that.

Many doctors have done this with great success. Dr. Robert Garrison in Ohio emails us with his feedback: "I've just hired a new hygienist. You did it again. She watched the first four sessions of the online course and her production today was $2,500."

Watching the online sessions have proven to be incredibly helpful to new hygienists.

Three Roles in Hygiene

When we train hygienists, we talk about maximizing their three critical roles:

- Periodontal therapist
- Preventive therapist

- Patient treatment advocate

It takes a long time to get a hygienist comfortable with operating under those three critical roles.

Before a hygienist gets to a level of high-performance, it can take a number of months, if not an entire year sometimes. There's a lot to know. There's a lot to learn.

Apply the idea of the 3-3-3 system (as described previously) to help guide them through becoming highly proficient.

Expectations for Progress

Expectations for production growth are unique to each practice. It depends on a few different factors:

- What is your past history?

- What model are you running?

- What resources are available to the hygienist?

    - If they have access to online courses, the goal should be different than if they're just trying to generate productivity growth on their own. That's going to take longer.

- Are your systems functioning at a high level?

- Is there a decent schedule for the provider?

All these factors need to be taken into account to make sure your expectations are realistic.

Creating Production Goals on a Timeline

It's not a bad idea to set expectations. For example, you could tell your hygienist:

- Within 30 days, we'd like your production average to be x.

- Within three months we'd like your production average to be y.

- After six months, we'd like your production average to be z.

It's even more effective if the new provider is involved in setting those goals.

- Ask the questions: "Where would you like to see your hourly productivity at in 30 days? Where would you like to be in six months? Where would you like to be after three months?"

- Like we always say, "People will support what they help create."

Comfort, Completeness and Speed

Comfort, completeness and speed — all three of these are important to patients. If you have one and not the other two, you're not going to be very effective.

- **Comfort is most important.** Hygienists and dentists who hurt people will end up not having many people to take care of.

   It doesn't matter if you have the best dentist in the world. If you have a hygiene provider that's hurting your patients, you're not going to have very many patients left.

People will walk. They'll disappear. They won't necessarily tell you. They silently leave.

- **Speed matters to patients more than ever.** They want it done as quickly as it can be done well. They don't want it done poorly, but they don't want to sit there all day either.

One of the biggest changes over the past few years is the lifestyle that our patients have. They are on the go. They are in the express lane. They want everything instantly. They don't want to be in the chair for two hours during a visit.

Dr. Meis:

We had two fantastic assistants in our office go back to school and become hygienists.

I posed the question to them, "How important was the patient's comfort in your training?"

Sadly, both of them said, "Not important at all."

Completeness was the only aspect of their training. Speed and comfort were unimportant.

Putting Hygienists Around Higher-Producing Hygienists

At our events, we regularly put a room full of people together who have similar struggles and challenges. They hear those who have already been there, done that and overcome it.

They realize, "If they can do it, so can I."

They're motivated when they see their peers and others accomplishing a $3,000 production day.

They ask specific questions about how it's possible.

There is so much value putting together groups of like-minded individuals who all want to improve.

Dr. Meis:

We recently had two hygienists who were with us before as dental assistants; they've only been licensed for three weeks and both have knocked on the door of $3,000.

Since they've worked in dentistry with their hands and in the mouth for many years, their speed is better than you would expect three weeks into practicing.

That said, yesterday one of them did $2,894. The other has been way up there as well.

All you have to do is to create the systems and then plug the right people in. Great systems make it easy for somebody to quickly be able to hit those numbers.

Hiring Associate Doctors

The End Game

So many doctors hire an associate without having a clear understanding of where their practice is going long-term.

Before you have an associate doctor, have it worked out.

Depending what your end game is, you're going to look for and attract different people.

You're going to be attracting completely different types of associates depending on your expectations.

It's better to clarify their opportunities in advance as opposed to having them get there and be disappointed because they had unrealistic expectations based on what you were offering.

Examples of the End Game

- **Burnout of practice.** As the doctor, you work and you practice. As you get older, you don't want to practice as much so you're not open as many hours. Your practice slowly and progressively goes downhill. When you go to sell it, you won't get very much because your practice isn't worth very much anymore.

- **Fizzle out.** As the doctor, you hire an associate, and then you start working less. Over time, the associate works more than you, then you just "fizzle out" as time goes by. If that's your strategy, you should have an associate who's going to be okay with that. Not all of them will be.

• **Other strategy.** The doctor gets all the crown, bridge and the cosmetics. The associate doctor gets all the simple operative and all the children. If that's your strategy, you should communicate that to the potential associate. Otherwise, they'll get into the practice and won't feel very satisfied.

Expect potential doctors to ask, "Can I become an owner?"

• Think about it thoroughly before you answer that question. It's going to be a very common question among associate candidates.

• There are many answers to that. For many doctors, their impression of "Is there going to be ownership?" is: "Are we going to be partners?" or "Am I going to buy you out?"

• Those are just two of the options with ownership. There are many more.

Having an understanding of your End Game is essential.

Know Your Numbers

Just like the delivery model in hygiene, how do you even know you're in need of an associate doctor if you're not aware of what your numbers are?

We see practices turn away patients and still say, "I'm good. I haven't gotten to the point where I need an associate."

It is far more frequent that someone has a significant capacity blockage when it comes to the doctor and they don't know it than there is a problem with demand and they don't know it.

Capacity is often one of the problems. That's why knowing your numbers is so important.

Potential associate doctors come in prepared to ask questions. Those questions are often on numbers.

- You have to remember you're selling yourself to the associate, just like they are selling themselves to you.

- If you're unprepared to answer some simple questions on numbers, it makes you not look like a great manager.

- Associate doctors come to your practice for your management help. If you know your numbers, they'll have significant confidence in your ability to manage.

We once interviewed an associate doctor. During the initial interview, she asked fantastic questions. Then, she sent a follow-up email with a whole string of numerical questions.

We were so impressed she had the insight to ask great questions about the numbers: new patients, staff turnover, reactivation systems, active patient bases, and insurance.

What was even more refreshing is we keep track of all of those metrics, so we were competent in providing the answers to those questions.

We don't know if she has the resources to totally understand the answers, but the fact that she asked them means she has studied up on what she should ask. It tells us she's put some time and effort in developing herself. The fact that we were prepared to answer her questions says we're a good place to consider.

Compensation Model for Associate Doctors

Some practices we work with pay their associates 40% of production while others pay 25%. It's all over the map. It is somewhat regional although not entirely.

Before attracting applicants, have a clear understanding of what you can do based on your own expense structure: What you can do, and what you can't do. Don't wait for the last minute to decide.

Don't just accept the compensation the potential associate requests:

- Heading down that road is going to be painful for you.

- Just because somebody wants more, doesn't mean you have to say yes.

- We don't know anyone who works hard, cares about their job, and does a great job that doesn't want more compensation. We all do. It's just part of the human nature of motivated people.

Have a clear-cut idea of what your compensation model is.

Delivery System for Associate Doctors

This is similar to what we talked about with the hygienists. There are quite a few questions to answer:

- Is this doctor going to be working with one assistant, two assistants or more?

- Is this doctor going to be working in one room, two rooms or more?

- Is this doctor going to be working 6 A.M.–9 A.M. and 4 P.M.–9 P.M. every day?

- Is this doctor going to be working 8:30 A.M.–3 P.M., so that their children can be dropped off at school and be picked up on the way home?

Prepare to be asked about your patients. How many new patients are you seeing? How many am I going to get? If the answer is "You get only the ones I don't want" or "You're not going to get any, you'll have to go out and find your own", then, that's not going to be very attractive to an associate doctor.

Make those kinds of decisions ahead of time. If you can communicate that to potential candidates, you can very quickly weed out many applicants who aren't going to fit with what your plan is.

Associate Readiness Check List

Readiness comes in three categories: Demand, Capacity and Emotional Preparedness.

Demand

1. Do you have enough new patient flow to feed an associate?

If you don't have more new patients than you can take care of, you're not ready. Associate doctors will go through more new patients than you do.

Most associates are young, so they are just like you were at their age. They have the same skills you did. They can't explain and sell treatment as well as you can. They can't produce it as fast as you can either.

Associates generally are not going to draw as many new patients as you do. They're not going to bring patients with them. They're looking to you to provide them a new patient flow.

They will go through more new patients. You have to accept that as part of the deal. You have to have the demand in place to feed that.

Having Enough New Patients

Make sure you have an adequate number of new patients.

If there isn't a good new patient flow beyond what the current doctors can see, you're not ready for an associate. Period.

In our experience, the owner-doctor always has a much higher case average per new patient than the associate doctor. It's often double. In order to reach the same production, the associate is going to need twice the number of new patients.

Associates fail when there is not an adequate number of new patients. Associates come in to the practice and they're not busy. There's not enough work to do, so they twiddle their thumbs. When they have lots of free time to think about how unhappy they are, that's when they move on. It's simple: People who are busy and productive are much happier.

2. Are you willing to improve your own marketing skills?

If the answer is no, you've got a problem. You probably don't have twice as many new patients coming as you can take care of. So, you've got to ramp up your new patient attraction skills (especially since the associate's going to use more than you).

3. Are you willing to increase your own marketing budget?

Your marketing budget feeds one doctor. You have to increase your marketing budget to feed two. It's got to be higher.

4. Do you have a positive track record of improving new patient flow with marketing?

We know practices that have tried everything for marketing, but their market is so competitive that marketing doesn't really draw more new patients.

- If the competition is incredibly fierce and you have a high dentist population ratio, this may not be possible.

If you don't have a positive track record of being able to do this, you're not ready for an associate.

You can put an associate in a distant location where the dentist population ratio is not so bad, but now you're managing a doctor at a different site. This causes its own problems.

- You're not there. So, you don't know what's happening. If they aren't in the same building, they will develop their own systems by chance and by luck (like we probably all did when we first started). That won't work very well.

Capacity

Do you have enough capacity to support an associate?

Most practices, in one way or another, are out of capacity.

Are you willing to face the capacity issues that you have to resolve in order to have enough capacity to support an associate?

Before you're ready for an associate, your team has to be good at same-day treatment.

In most practices, same-day treatment is what feeds the associate for the first few months or year.

Our practice does $3,000–$9,000 a day of same-day treatment. This treatment was not on the books. It came out of Hygiene or walk-ins.

It is a tremendous pool that most practices don't take advantage of.

Your associate has to practice somewhere to treat patients.

Here's the thing dentists don't understand—they've got to have a place to practice.

If you think you're going to get an associate who's going to work evenings and weekends so that you can have a 9–5 job, that's unrealistic. If you're in a very competitive area, you can get someone to do that for a while, but that isn't setting that person up for success.

You need to have some place for them to treat patients. There's got to be room or time.

Another frequent mistake is that the associate doctor gets the rooms nobody wants with old or broken equipment, or both.

Putting the associate in that room isn't setting them up for success.

Are you able to expand hours and days of operation?

If you don't have enough treatment rooms at the same time, you can expand hours and days of operation.

We've done this multiple times in our growth curve. We ran split shifts. We had a 7 A.M.–1 P.M. and a 1 P.M.–7 P.M. shift. We've also done Saturdays. Saturdays are always great for patients.

Does your facility allow you to do this? Some professional locations don't allow offices to be open during certain times. Is your team mentally prepared for this schedule? Are your team members able to work those hours?

You're going to be more likely to succeed if you have a team leader managing the practice.

If you're going to personally manage the associates, that's going to take time. It's going to take longer but its great for owner doctors to do.

The associate is going to need more time developing and understanding values and culture of your practice.

There's going to be many discussions about where they didn't live up to standards.

The associate doctor will often ask specific questions like, "Can you look at this x-ray?"

If you try to manage other team members and develop a new doctor, either you'll run out of time or it'll affect your personal productivity. If it's taking your time out of the chair, it's going to be a bust on profitability.

If it affects your personal productivity, your practice profitability will suffer. Avoid that at all costs.

Are you willing to hire additional team members?

You'll need additional team members if you have an additional doctor. There's no question.

If you're not in a place to hire an additional assistant, maybe two, and an additional front office person, you're not going to have the capacity to make that person successful.

Emotional Preparedness

Are you emotionally prepared? This is the tough one.

Are you willing to take on the responsibility of doing what you can do to help that associate succeed?

If you're not, you're not ready.

Are you willing to do for the associate what no one did for you?

Owner doctors, in frustration, often complain, "Nobody did that for me." That's crying over spilled milk. It doesn't matter what somebody did for you. It's about what you're going to do to help that associate be successful.

Are you willing to give a greater share of the new patients to the associate?

They're going to need more than you are. They need to have enough to get started and get their speed improved. Every dentist was slow when they got out of dental school. We all got faster over time.

Associate doctors are largely young. Their speed is going to take time to develop.

Are you willing to give the associate your best chair side assistant?

If the answer is no, you're not ready.

This often makes people nauseous to think about. This doesn't have to be permanent, but it's certainly the best resource for moving the associate along in the training continuum.

Your best assistant will help mold the doctor. They are assertive enough to say privately and out of the way, "That's not how we do things here. Here's how we handle that."

Often associate doctors understand the technical aspects of dentistry but don't understand the people element of dentistry very well.

Your new associate doctor needs to become an excellent communicator. An assertive assistant will tell them how they can be better and how they can improve.

Having an assistant who is very good at those things and is assertive enough to give honest and direct feedback to the associate is really important.

From patients' perspectives, it's a good transition. The doctor is brand-new, but they have an existing relationship with the assistant, and they're very comfortable with them.

Are you willing to make less income temporarily while the associate ramps up?

If you're not willing to accept that, you're not emotionally prepared for an associate.

When you give them some of the new patients you're using, you're going to have a temporary dip in income. It will go up, but there'll be a temporary dip.

So, Are You Ready?

- If you can answer "yes" to all of those questions, you're ready.

- If you can answer yes to two-thirds of them, you're ready.
- If you can only answer "yes" to a handful, you're not ready.

We can guarantee you that having an associate doctor, over the first six months, is not going to reduce your stress.

We can guarantee you that because there's a period of development. There's a period where your team has to buy in to that person. Expect members to come up to you and say, "Can I talk to you?" then break bad news.

Initially, it's going to be more work and more stress.

It takes time to work through those things, but you can. If everyone has the same good intention, you do get through the stress, but it's not without work.

Set Them Up for Success

Associate doctors are young and inexperienced. They don't know your treatment philosophies, and they're not ingrained in the values of your practice.

How Associates are Treated Traditionally

You hire a new assistant, who is inexperienced, to work with an inexperienced associate in the crappy rooms. That's not setting that person up for success. If you do that, they're less likely to be successful.

If you do that, years from now you're going to be at a dental meeting telling other doctors that associate-ships don't work.

They do work, but they don't work the way you did them.

The Right Mindset

What we're trying to do is set up a framework and a mindset that's going to be the most likely to be successful for you and, just as importantly, successful for the associate.

If you take on an associate, there's a certain amount of responsibility you have to that person, just like all team members. You're taking on the responsibility of helping that person develop.

Learn About Their Past and Future

Opportunity or Security

During the process of hiring associate doctors, determine if they're looking for security or if they're looking for opportunity.

Do they ask lifestyle and security-based questions?

- How much vacation time am I going to get?

- How many hours a week am I going to have to work?

- Will I get the full lunch hour?

Or do they ask opportunity questions:

- How many new patients will I see?

- Do we each have our own patients?

- Are they everyone's patients?

- Do we accept insurance? Do we do emergency care?

- Can I become an owner?

- I enjoy surgery. Does the current doctor enjoy doing surgery? Do you refer much surgery out?

When you have somebody asking the latter type of questions, you can tell they're looking for opportunity, not security.

Past Experiences

If they've had previous employment, ask them to tell you about it:

- What worked about it?

- What was really great about it?

- What did they enjoy about it?

- What would they have changed if they could have?

Asking questions like these draws out a lot from people. For example, if you ask, "What did you enjoy about your past experiences?" and the response is, "Nothing. There was not a good thing about that place." Now, you've got an idea of the attitude of that person.

Some associate doctors may just be unhappy. They may go from one bad experience to the next. If you hire them, you're going to be their next bad experience because they're determined to have one.

Past experiences, in that way, are a good indicator of future success.

Past Productivity

Past productivity, on the other hand, is not always a reliable indicator.

If the associate doctors have a very high number, that's a good indicator.

If they don't have a high number, it doesn't necessarily tell you what you think it does.

Many times, the associates weren't given the opportunity to be productive or they weren't in the right environment with the right systems.

We routinely double but usually triple past productivity because of our systems, our team and all the things we have in place to help get people there.

Compare Philosophies

It's great to have a conversation about procedures and philosophies because not everyone has the same philosophy.

For example, if you think amalgam is the best material that's ever been made in dentistry, you'll find there are some dentists who disagree with you on that. They don't think it's a good material at all.

If you're going to be working with somebody, your philosophies and your ideas about different procedures and materials need to be very close.

It doesn't have to be exactly the same, but it needs to be very close. Otherwise, it will confuse patients, and confused patients run for the door.

Having some conversations about procedures and philosophies ahead of time is helpful.

Ability to Work as a Team Member

It's vital that associate doctors see themselves as part of the team.

Whether you're a doctor, hygienist, or an assistant, it's of utmost important to have a team mindset.

The need to be willing and able to do whatever it takes to get what needs to be done done is essential. Everyone is working for the common good of the practice. They see that "we are all in this together."

Training

After You've Hired the New Associate

For training, we have associates spend their first six days doing every job in the office.

Often, it's a week or longer before they start seeing patients.

It's everything from reviewing the schedules on how we schedule to reviewing the new patient process, the practice management software, how we do noting, what we are doing for marketing, and so on. Truly, associates learn every position in the practice.

A lot is gained from training associates using this process:

1. **It helps them to meet the people in the office and get to know them better.** It helps them get off on the right foot with the entire team because it gives them an opportunity to get to know them. It's an opportunity for the team to see their focus, interest, and drive.

2. **It helps them to understand how the systems work and how they all interlink.** If one person in one area doesn't follow their part of the system, they see how it screws everything up. They see it takes a lot of people to really make this practice work and work well.

3. **It begins their process of being another member of the team.** "I'm doing whatever it takes. If it's answering the

phone, if it's collecting payments, I'm doing whatever needs to be done. "

4. **It lets them know that for everything they do with each patient, there's so much that happens behind the scenes.** They see we're going to do our best to make sure they can keep doing their best.

5. **They understand they're going to be held accountable. They have to be approved when they work.** They're going to sit there and won't be able to do dentistry until they learn what they need to learn. For instance, in the front office, they have to be approved by the area's team leader that they understand the systems and are ready to move on.

Associates don't expect this kind of training. They're surprised because they think they're just going to dive in and do dentistry. It's been extremely valuable to have it not happen that way.

Spending Time With Other Doctors

Another piece of the training is having the associate doctors spend time with the other doctors in the office.

So, if it was a two-doctor office, it would be the two doctors sitting down and going over treatment, cases and frustrations. They just have conversations about dentistry.

Dentistry is an extremely isolating profession. One of the most profoundly satisfying things about working in a practice with multiple doctors is the ability to do this.

The support and understanding of other people who do the same job and with the same frustrations can sometimes be the only thing that keeps you from pulling your hair out. It's a wonderful thing about having another doctor in the office.

Use doctor-doctor time to discuss cases. If there's a complicated or difficult case, talk through it as a group.

Discuss a "treatment mismatch." This is where one doctor diagnosed a problem, had X treatment designed for that and the other doctor thought Y treatment would have been better.

Those "treatment mismatches" decrease over time. They get smaller and smaller (as long as everyone discusses it with an open mind).

Discuss quality issues. Doctors have an obligation to patients to make sure everyone is doing good quality work.

If there are things that aren't working like they ought to be, we have those conversations as well.

When you have those kinds of conversations with someone who knows you, cares about you and is committed to making the practice be as good as it could possibly be, it makes those difficult conversations go very smoothly.

Doing Everything the Same Way

Dr. Meis: We don't do it my way, do we?
Heather: We do not.

Dr. Meis: We don't do it your way?
Heather: We don't do it my way.

Dr. Meis: What way do we do it?
Heather: We do it the best way.

We all do things in the same way. We use the same materials. We use the same techniques.

It's not 100% the same, but it's close; close enough for any doctor to work with any assistant in our office. They know what I'm going to do because we do it that close.

Doing Things "Our Way"

If we find a better way, that'll then become "our way" and we'll all do it that way.

- I can name numerous changes, both in material and technique, we've all adopted because it was a better way.

- "Better" means it's higher quality, lower costs, faster or more comfortable.

- If we can make an improvement on two of those, we're going to make a change on it. It's that simple.

Getting Everyone on the Same Page

- It's not easy to do. You've to involve everyone and collect their input so that they can support what you decide upon.

- This takes time but the benefits from it are tremendous for efficiency, productivity, ease of training and use of our assistants.

What Happens If We Don't Do It the Same Way

- We have the same materials and equipment, so we don't need, for example, five different systems for doing Endo or 15 types of sutures.

Decide What's Going to be Useful and Always Have It

We decided on the instruments that are going to go on the cassette. That took a while, believe it or not. You'd think it would be a real easy decision, but it wasn't because you only have so many spots.

The Current Draft

What we end up deciding is then called the "current draft." We always refer to changes as the current draft. Just because we decide it's the best way today, it doesn't mean that's how it's always going to stay.

Anytime we want to make a change or implement a new system, that's how we present it to our team.

Change can be difficult. This is a really non-threatening and comforting way of saying, "If it doesn't work, it'll change again."

They know that if we find out there's a better, quicker, more efficient, more comfortable way of doing something, then we're certainly going to make another change—and it becomes our new current draft.

Using that terminology of the current draft makes people aren't as resistant because they know it's going to change again. You're not locking something in that's going to be there forever.

We strive for continuous development—progress not perfection.

Summary

While reading this you may have thought, "Oh! I probably stepped in it here." That's very common, but we really need to be careful and be more diligent than in the past.

Everything we discussed is really just treating people fairly, communicating directly, communicating with brutal honesty, doing it in as kind a manner as possible, doing it the same for everyone—and those are just good principles.

You're going to find you have a lot more consistency, a lot more happiness within the team, and it works a whole lot better if everyone's treated the same in a fair manner.

Appendix I: Creating a Dental Assisting School

One area we were having an extremely difficult time keeping fully staffed was dental assistants.

Our local community college educates dental assistants, but they don't educate enough. Less than 20 students graduate every year. This small pool is all we had to work with in all of Northwest Iowa. We're in a tri-state region, so a lot of these assistants were going to Nebraska and South Dakota as well.

We realized that if we were going to have a ready pool of prospective employees who were trained and a good fit, we needed to do more. Therefore, we started our own in-house dental assisting school.

Our dental assisting school is a non-traditional setting. It's an accelerated 10-week course.

- All of the bookwork is done online.

- Students spend 10 Saturdays in the practice doing hands-on clinical techniques such as radiography and impressions.

- Students aren't able to actually practice on real patients during that time, so they use Dexter mannequins.

- Once they graduate from this dental assisting school, they have some hoops to jump through with the board of examiners in our state. This proves they're capable, knowledgeable and can do their job in a safe way.

Our students generally are non-traditional: mothers and people who work full time. They work and attend school on the weekend. Often, they are more committed because they are taking it on as an extra in their already busy life.

Having a Birds-Eye View on Prospective Employees

The course allows us to have a bird's-eye view of prospective employees—our students.

It allows us to have an opportunity to get to know the students and know which ones we think would fit in well with our team.

We see a variety of factors, including:

- Who shows up on time

- Who asks great questions

- Who interacts well with other students

- Who scores highly on their tests and quizzes

Last time we counted, almost half of our team came from our own dental assisting school. It's not just clinical team members, it's administrative team members as well.

Team Involvement

The course is taught by our own team members.

It's a great opportunity for our own team to take a step to further develop themselves as people. It gives our own team an opportunity to teach others. This is extremely beneficial because, as many people attest, the teacher always learns more than the student.

They also see first-hand the people we have to choose from. They determine:

- Who are the people they're going to want to work with

- Who are the people they're going to want to add to our team

The associate doctors volunteer and rotate turns on Saturdays. There's instrument transfer, making the field, and so on.

That's been a really great way to get the entire team on board with expanding our team and really committing to making someone else's life so much better.

Developing the Assisting School

We hired a programmer to put all of the didactic material online. All the tests and quizzes are done online so their Saturday in the office is all hands-on with dental materials: radiography, impressions, polishing teeth, learning instruments' names, and so on.

We originally purchased the curriculum for the dental assisting school. Over time, we have changed it, adapted it, massaged it, and improved it. Today, you wouldn't even recognize the original. It's so much better now.

Today, some of the course trainers were students who had gone through the course.

Appendix II: Social Media and Electronic Communication

At Work

Statistics say over 700 billion minutes per month are spent on Facebook. Over 2.5 billion text messages are sent each day. That's an unfathomable amount of time. Obviously, some of it has to be taking place at work.

With blogs, email, Facebook and Twitter, there's a major blurring of the lines between what's private and personal in a professional space.

If you're going to punish the use of these types of media during work, you need to do it consistently and practice what you preach. No one should be on their Facebook page during working hours, not even doctors; it just sends the wrong message.

Remember, do it in a consistent manner and have it clearly defined in your policy manual that those are forbidden. If, for example, you allow them during break time, make sure it's clearly defined, consistently enforced and train your employees on what the policy is.

Define your policy on email exchange: Can it be of personal nature? Should it only be exchanged between people within the practice? What punishments should follow violations? How many times should you be warned? Is termination going to result for using work email for personal messages?

At Home

Social media use at home and what can be said about the practice publicly can be in the policy. Set a clear expectation for how much privacy is being afforded. Clarify if there is any expectation of privacy during your off hours.

For example, you could say, "If it has to do with the practice, other employees or patients, there is no expectation of privacy."

Due to the consequences, from wasting time to performance issues to disclosing confidential information, you must make it very clear in your policy manual. Explicitly state what will and will not be tolerated, and enforce it all the time in a consistent manner.

Former Employees

Protect yourself from what former employees may write. State in the policy that any and all information, confidential or otherwise, stays with the practice even when employees leave the practice and that they are not of liberty to disclose any information about the practice following their departure.

Beyond that, it becomes an issue of freedom of speech. Everyone's entitled to their own opinion. But if you have someone who is continuously spreading negative comments about the practice or about patients, that's a good time to have your attorney or HR resource write up a cease and desist letter.

Even the smallest things can offend patients or your current employees. There's only so much you can censor, but there's an awful lot that can be accomplished in taking the right measures to ask someone to stop.

Online communication doesn't have the same filters that are used in person. People are used to saying things online that wouldn't necessarily say in public. It's going to be an ongoing and difficult problem.

That said, some people are bent on burning bridges and don't know when to leave well enough alone. If a few negative Facebook posts are what it takes to end their frustration and move on, then in the grand scheme, it's fairly irrelevant. We'd rather have someone vent real quick about us online as opposed to seek advice from an employment lawyer.

Your Own Behavior Online

As a practice, you shouldn't post things about your employees or former employees that aren't of a positive nature. No good can come from that.

It's a two-way street, so each person has the expectation that their reputation will be held intact after the relationship ends. It should end without any need to comment publicly.

Appendix III: Continuing Education

Here are some additional experiences that are helpful for a hygiene provider as they progress.

In-Office Consultations

- We take great pride in providing a very powerful day that's a great experience, regardless of the level of experience of the hygiene providers you've got.

- It's helpful for practices who are trying to decide what model of hygiene they should run or what production-based compensation model they want to implement. They may have a fairly new team and they just want to facilitate results.

Seminars

We do a variety of seminars every year.

- The Backstage Pass event tours Dr. Meis' practice on a working day to see a high-level practice in action.

- We have a couple of topic-specific seminars:

o   If you want your hygiene department to be updated on the latest and greatest as far as periodontal treatments are concerned, we hold a seminar on that.

o   We hold seminars on a world-class experience, the new patient experience and case assessment.

Online Courses and DVDs

- There's no replacement for live training, but we have had very good results with online courses.

In a nutshell, we're committed to help develop dental teams with whatever their needs may be.

It just depends on what area you want to focus on. Once you know that, we can guide you in the right direction.

Dr. Meis:

I can tell you that our team has done an awful lot of additional experiences.

Each time they do, they come back more focused, their productivity goes up, and their energy about it goes up. They're passion for it goes up.

We all need, from time to time, a little injection of motivation to push our passion up again. The wear and tear of clinical dentistry sometimes wears us down a little bit.

So, having an experience with you and one of your coaches has been helpful for us to push that passion level back up.

Made in the USA
Monee, IL
23 January 2021